THIS IS FOR ELI AND ANYONE ELSE WHO HAS EVER BEEN TOLD THAT THEY ARE WEIRD FOR BEING WHO THEY ARE.

FOR THOSE WHO NEED TO LEARN BETTER. MAY THIS SERVE AS A KIND REMINDER THAT BEING MISUNDERSTOOD, BEING OUTSIDE THE BOX, STANDING OUT WHILE EVERYONE ELSE IS IN LINE DOES NOT MEAN SOMEONE IS WEIRD. IT MEANS THEY ARE AN INDIVIDUAL, A TRENDSETTER, SPECIAL, DESERVING OF RECOGNITION AND POSITIVE REINFORCEMENT. MAKE TIME TO BE KIND AND YOU WILL NEVER REGRET IT.

You looked at me confusingly and with a question on your mind, "Am I weird?!" you asked.

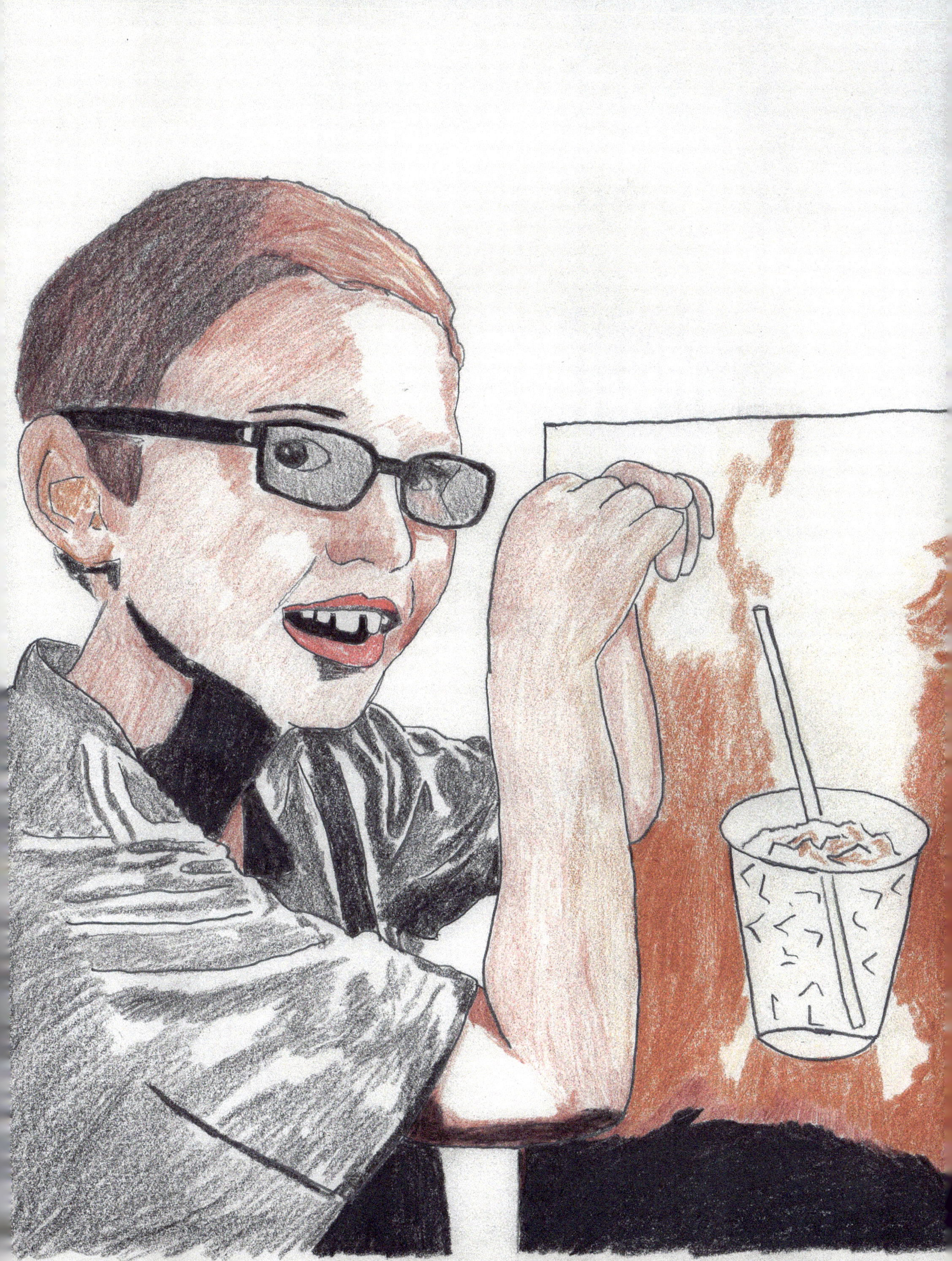

Yes child, you are not

typical, but you are

all my favorite

things.

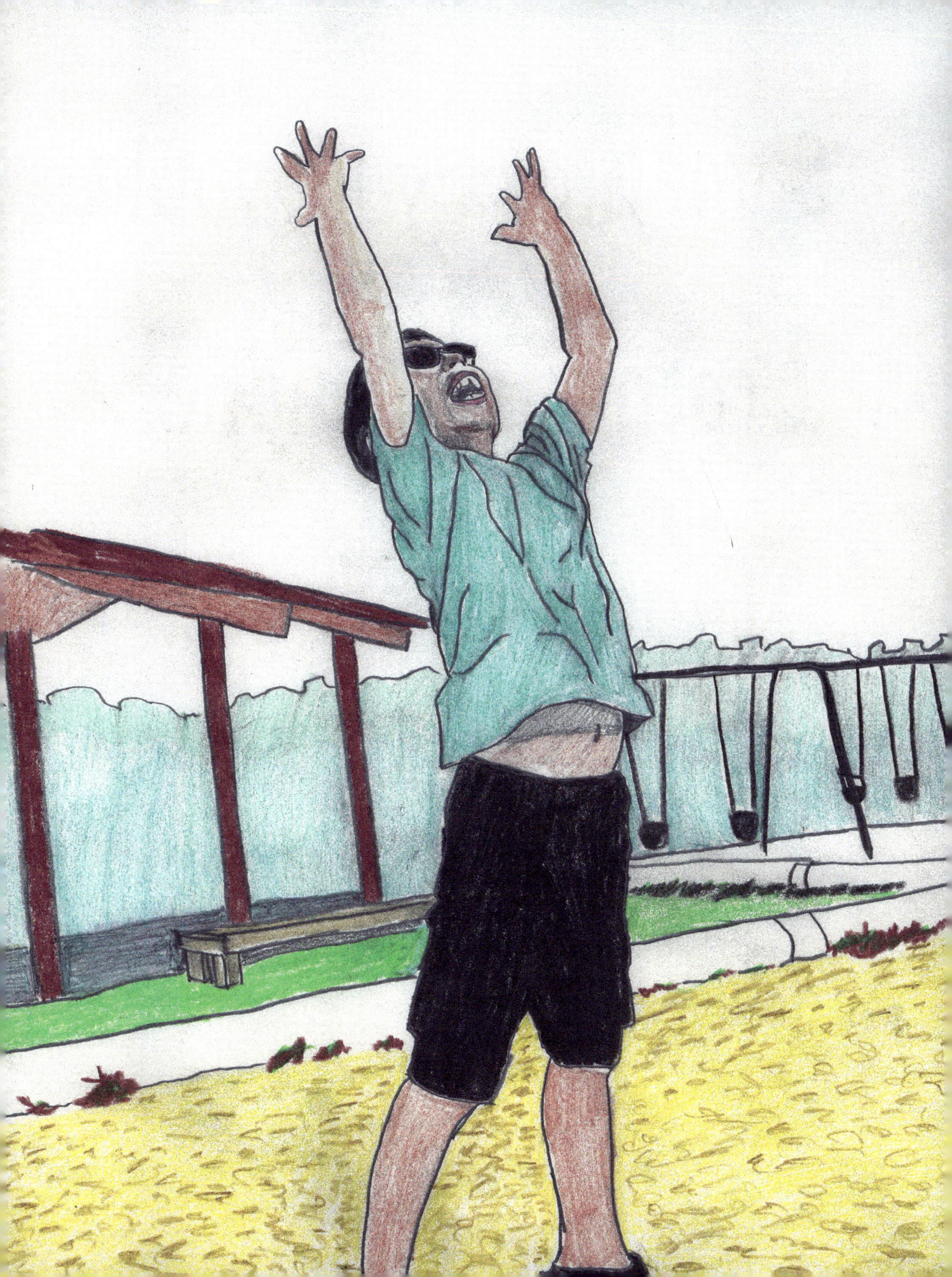

Sometimes you would

rather play alone

than with others.

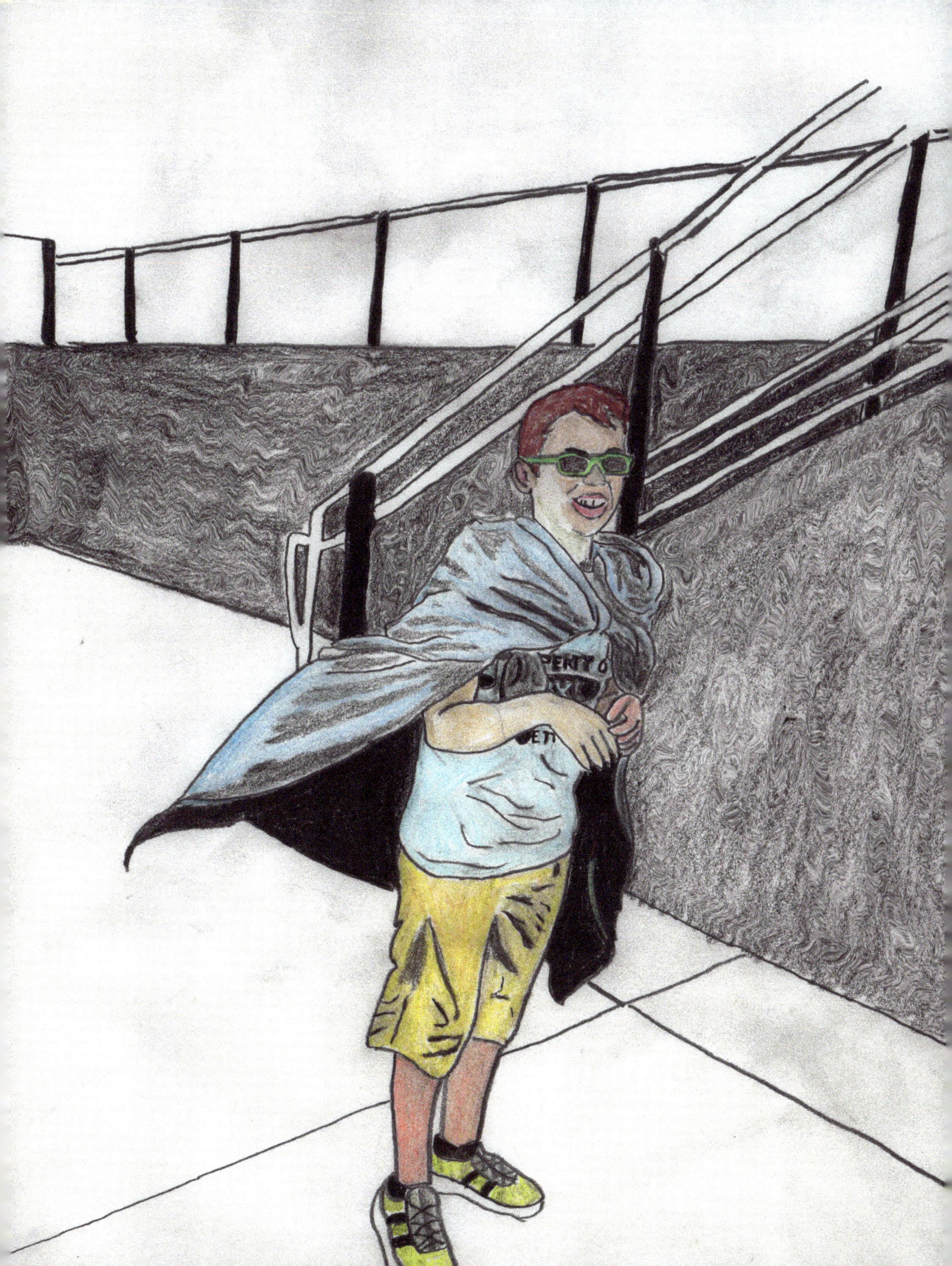

Sometimes you line

your toys up and get

mad if anyone tries

to move them.

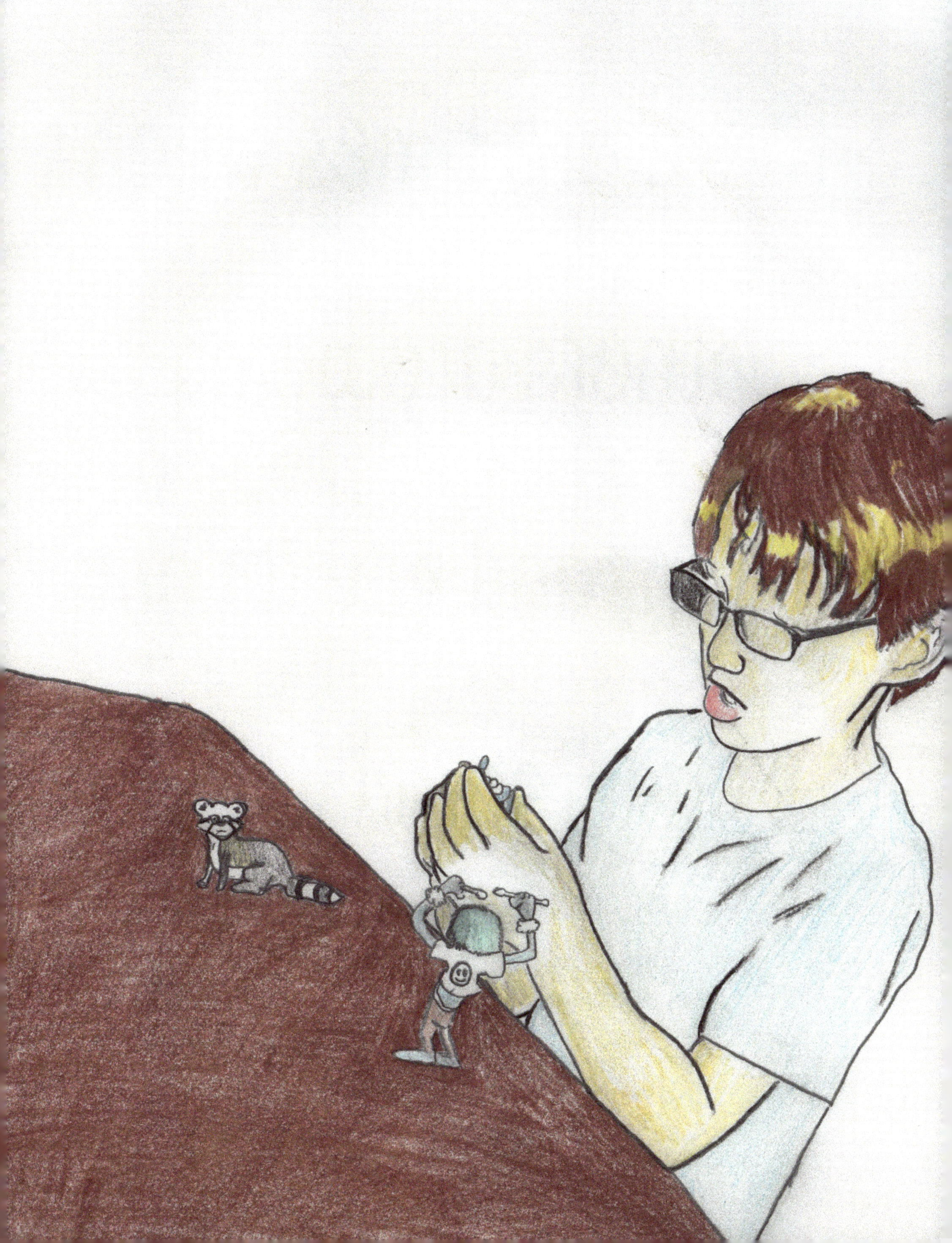

There are times when

others are being

mean, and you do not

understand why.

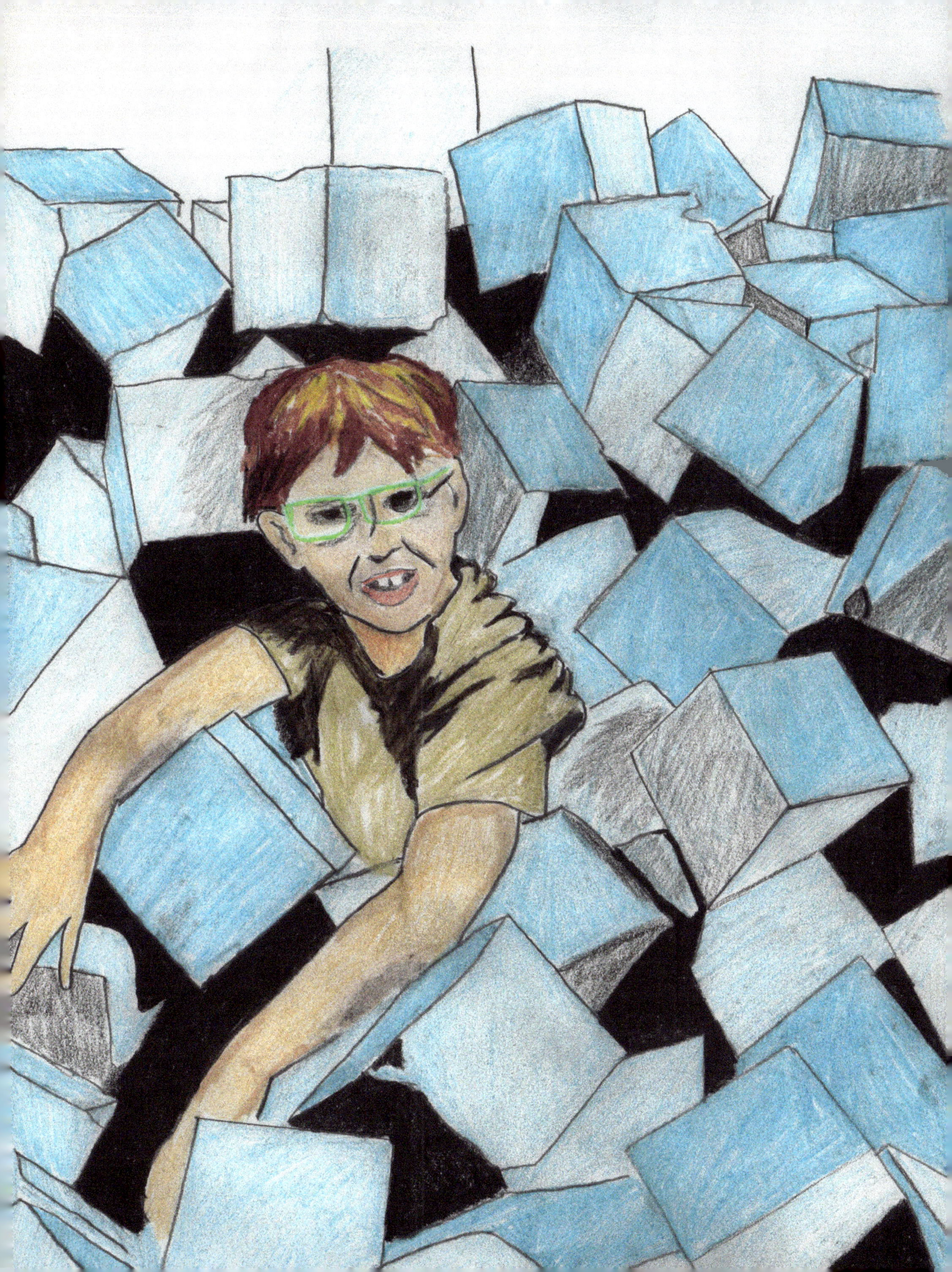

You can always see good in people. Some make that harder than others, but you find a way.

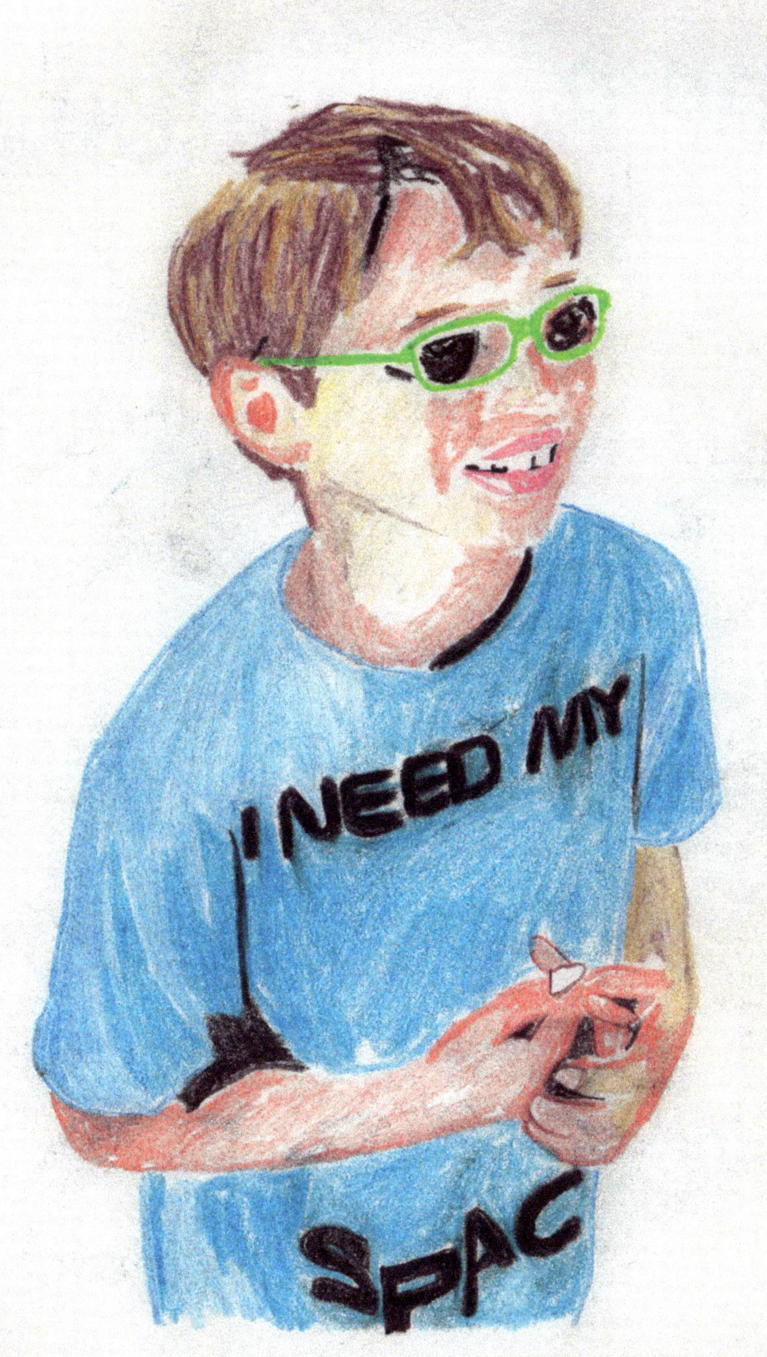

I NEED MY
SPAC

Words do not always

come easy when you

need to express how

you feel and that is

frustrating.

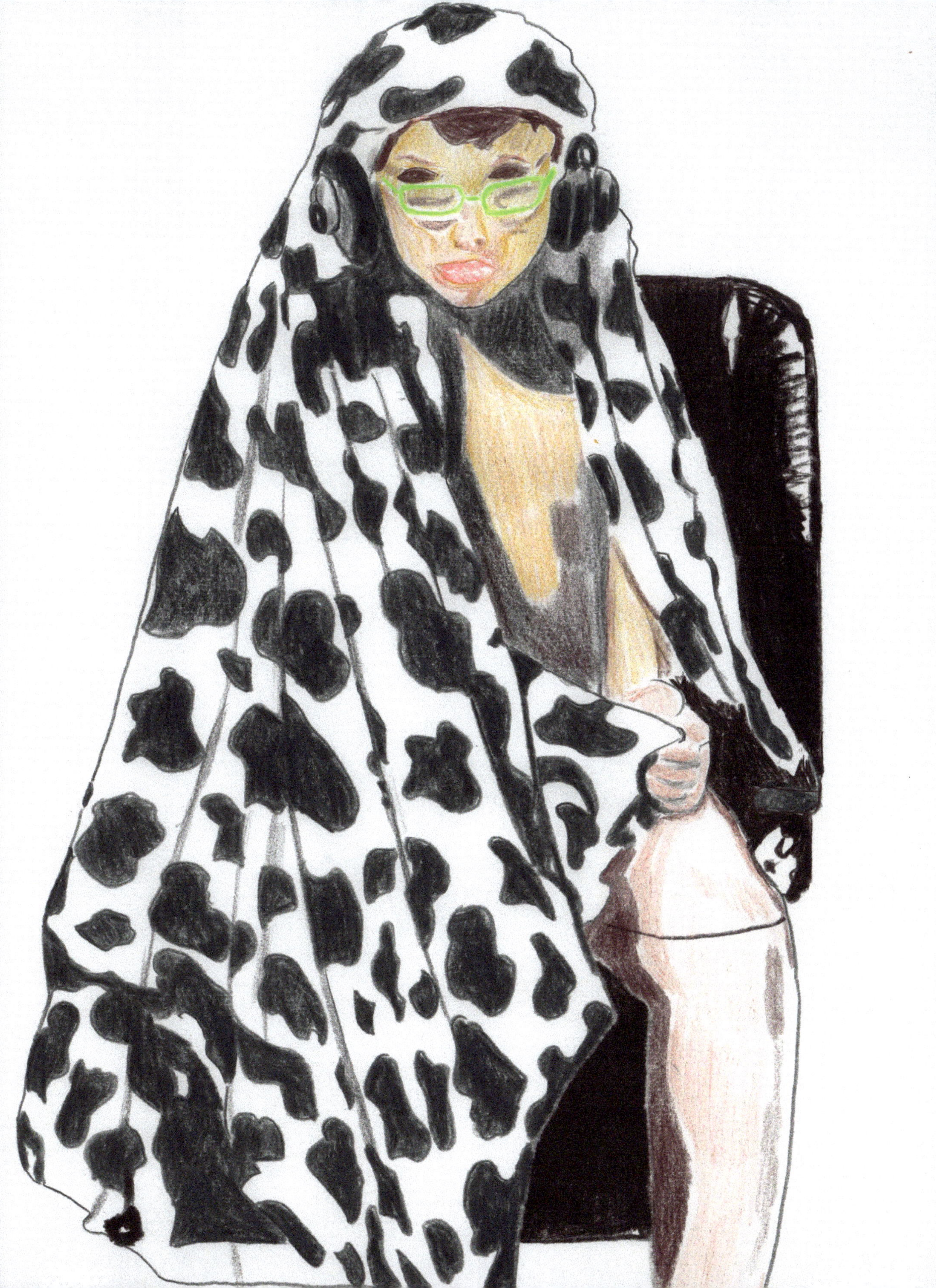

So many things you do are different. You have your own way to exist.

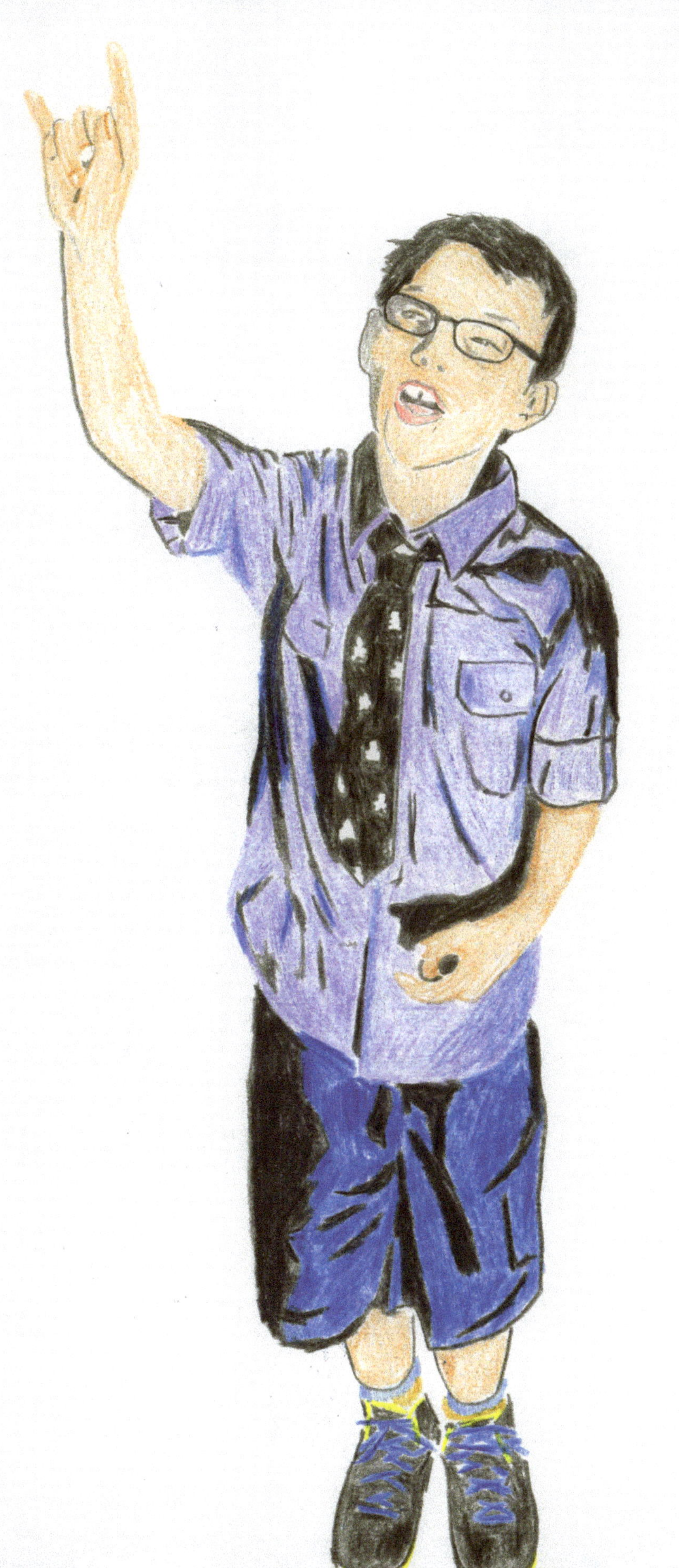

There are times when

you can only

physically express

yourself, and that is

okay too!

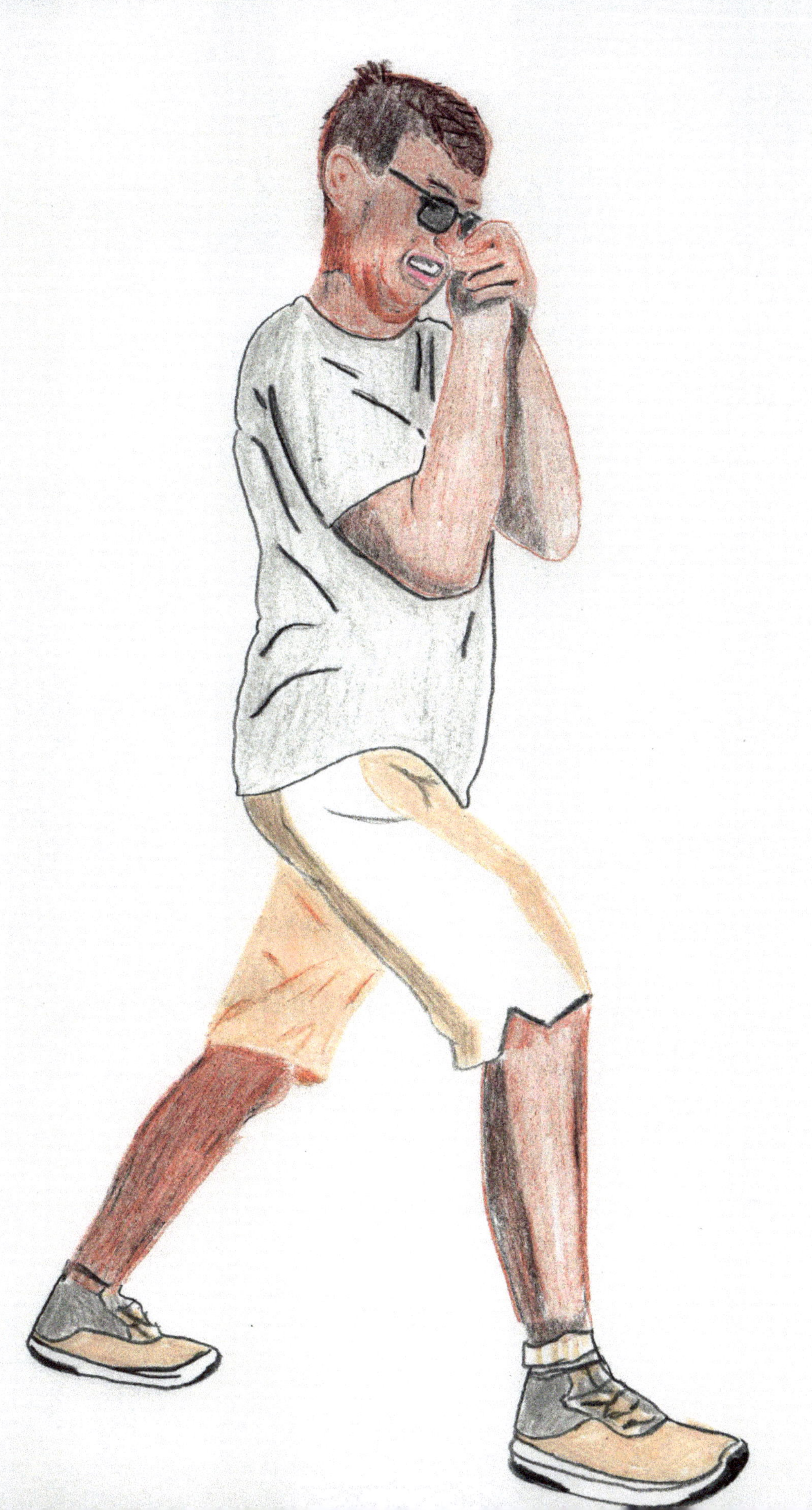

Loud noises can

bother you

sometimes and get

you overstimulated.

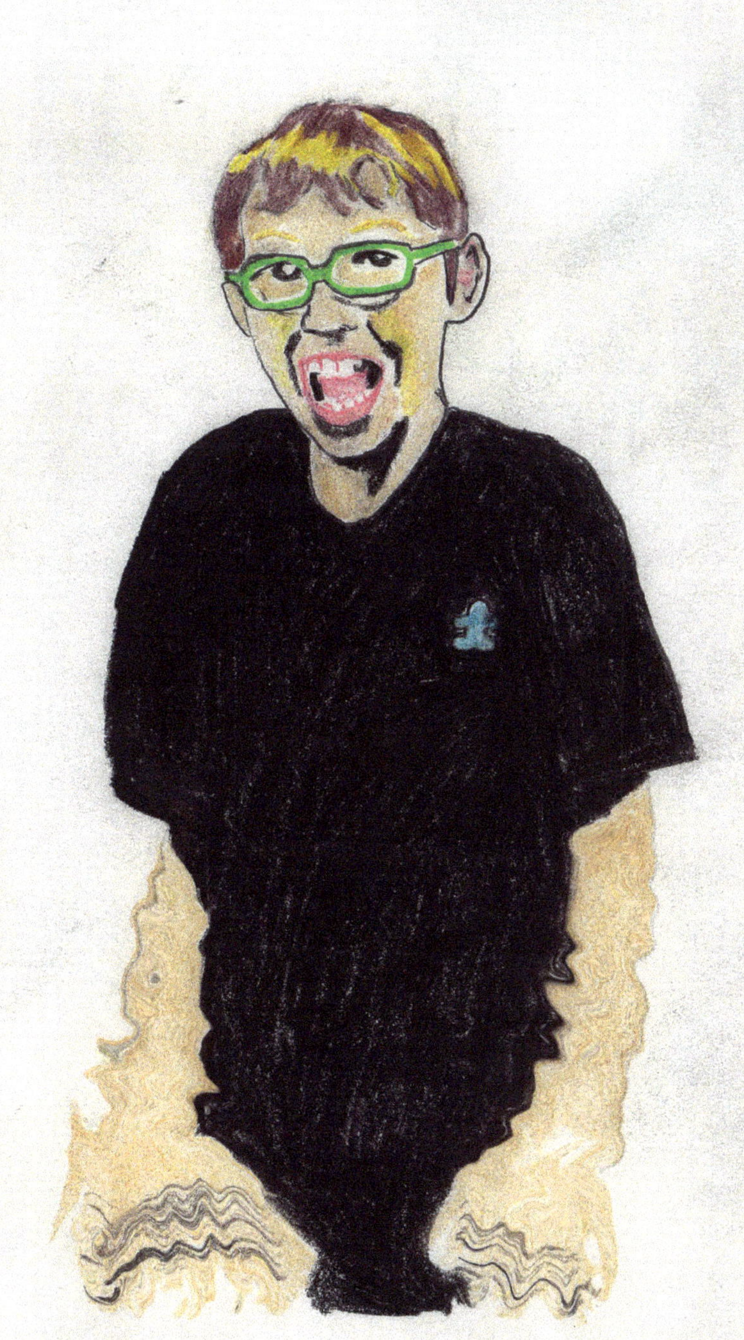

Sometimes you make

new food

combinations that

only you will eat.

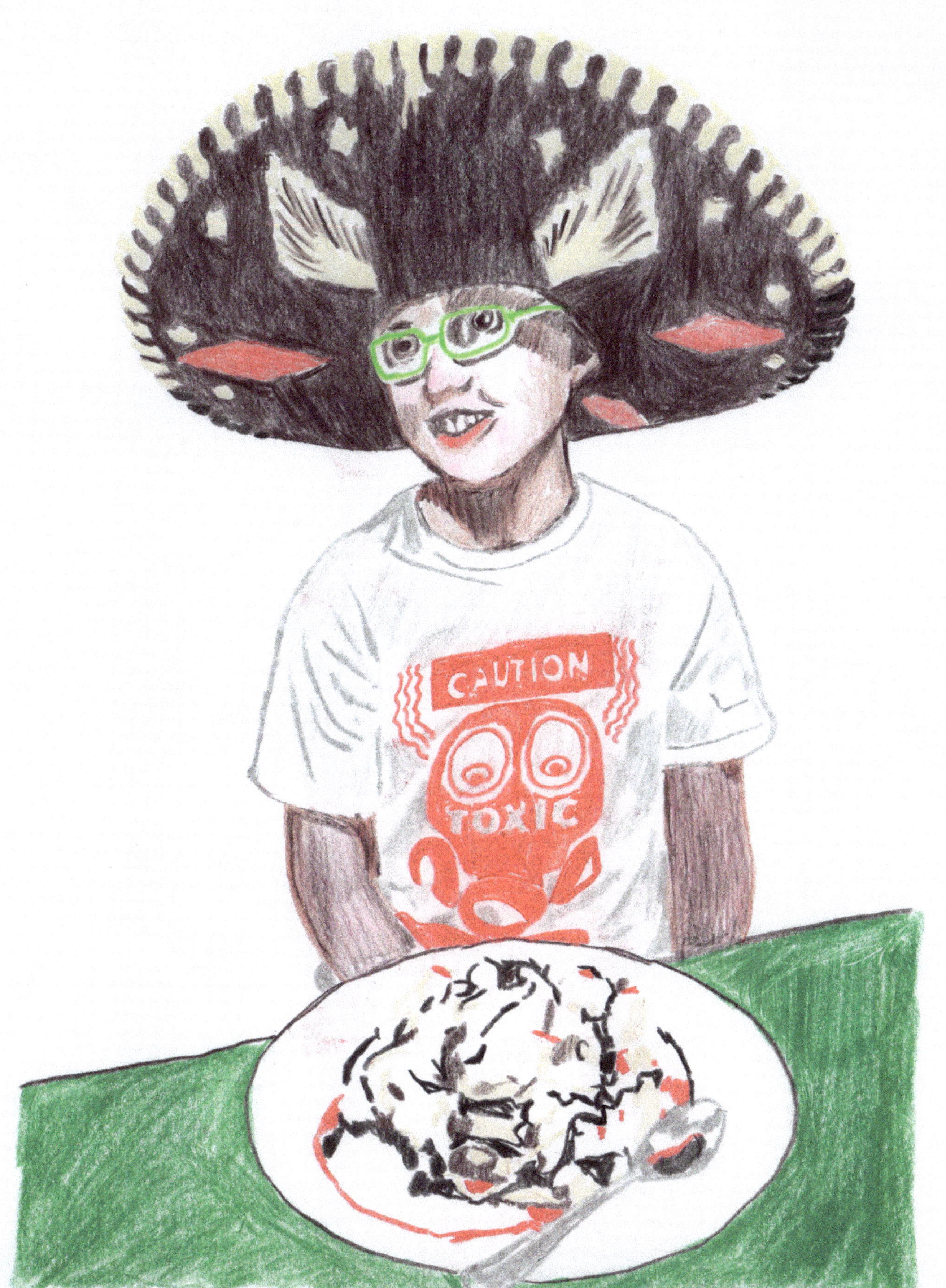
CAUTION
TOXIC

So, yes son you do things unlike anyone else.

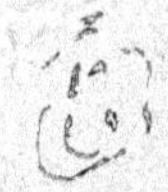

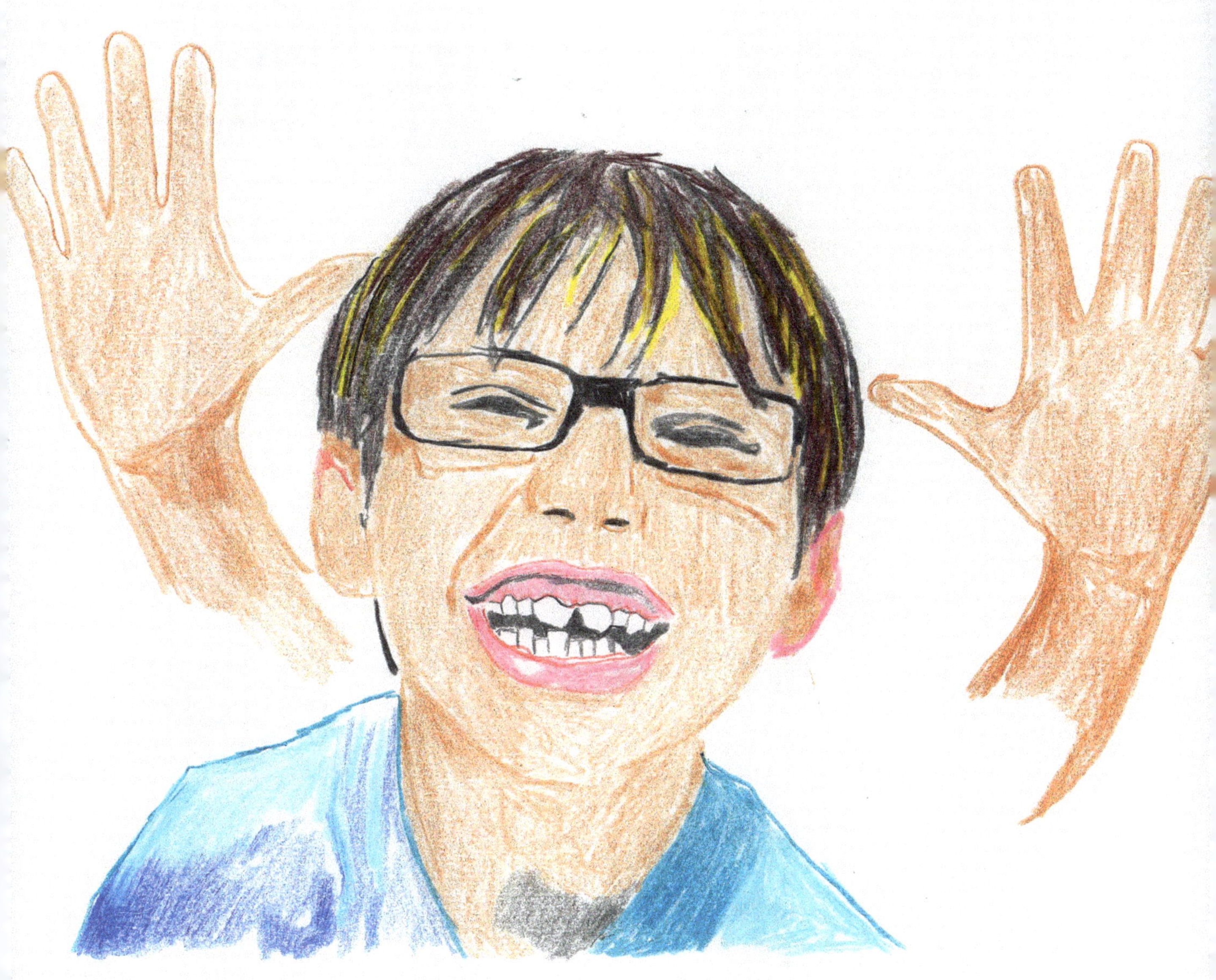

You do things unexpectedly at times and this can require a lot of patience.

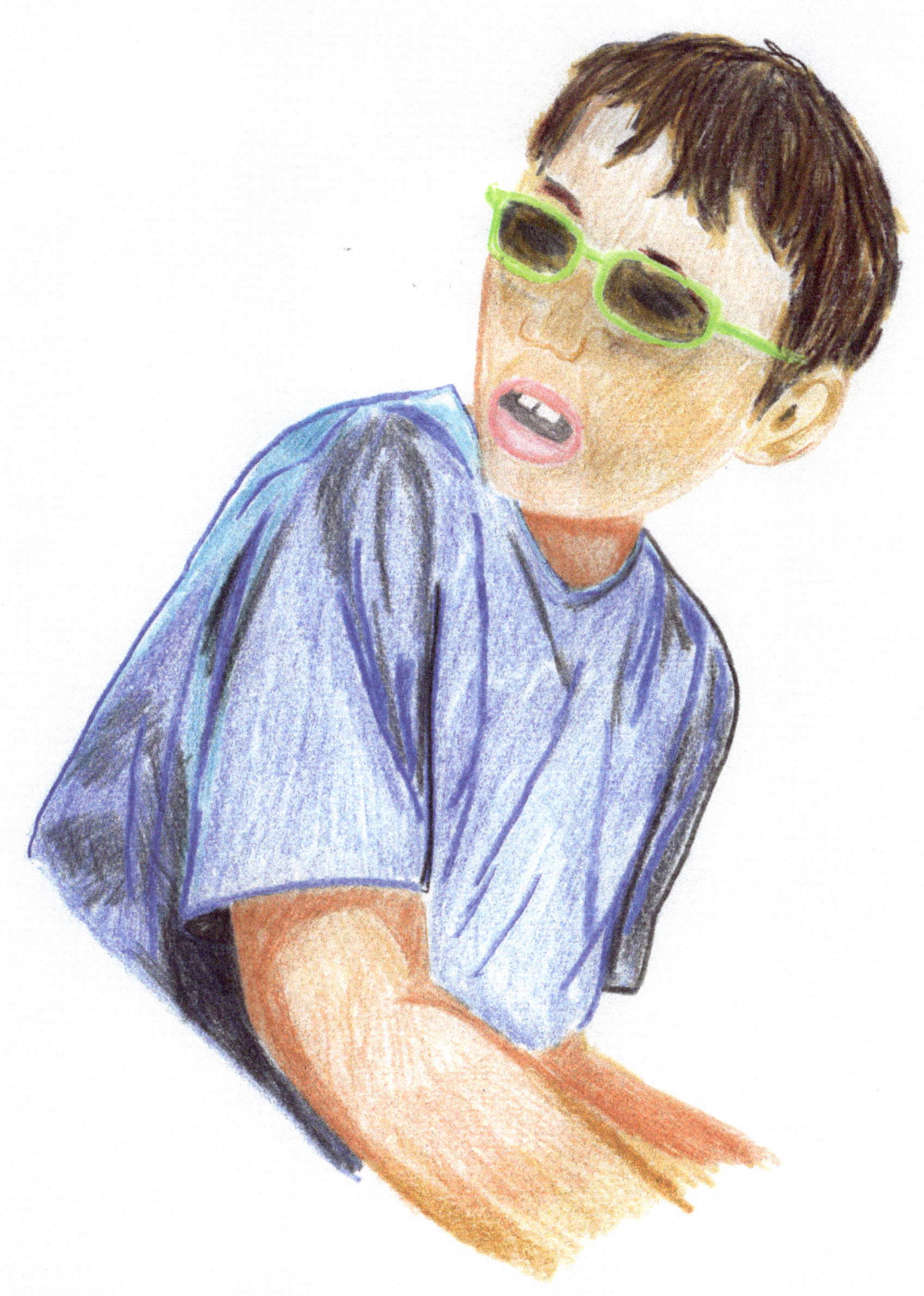

If this is what the world calls "weird" then I need you to know that this is something everyone could strive to be. Thank you for being YOU!

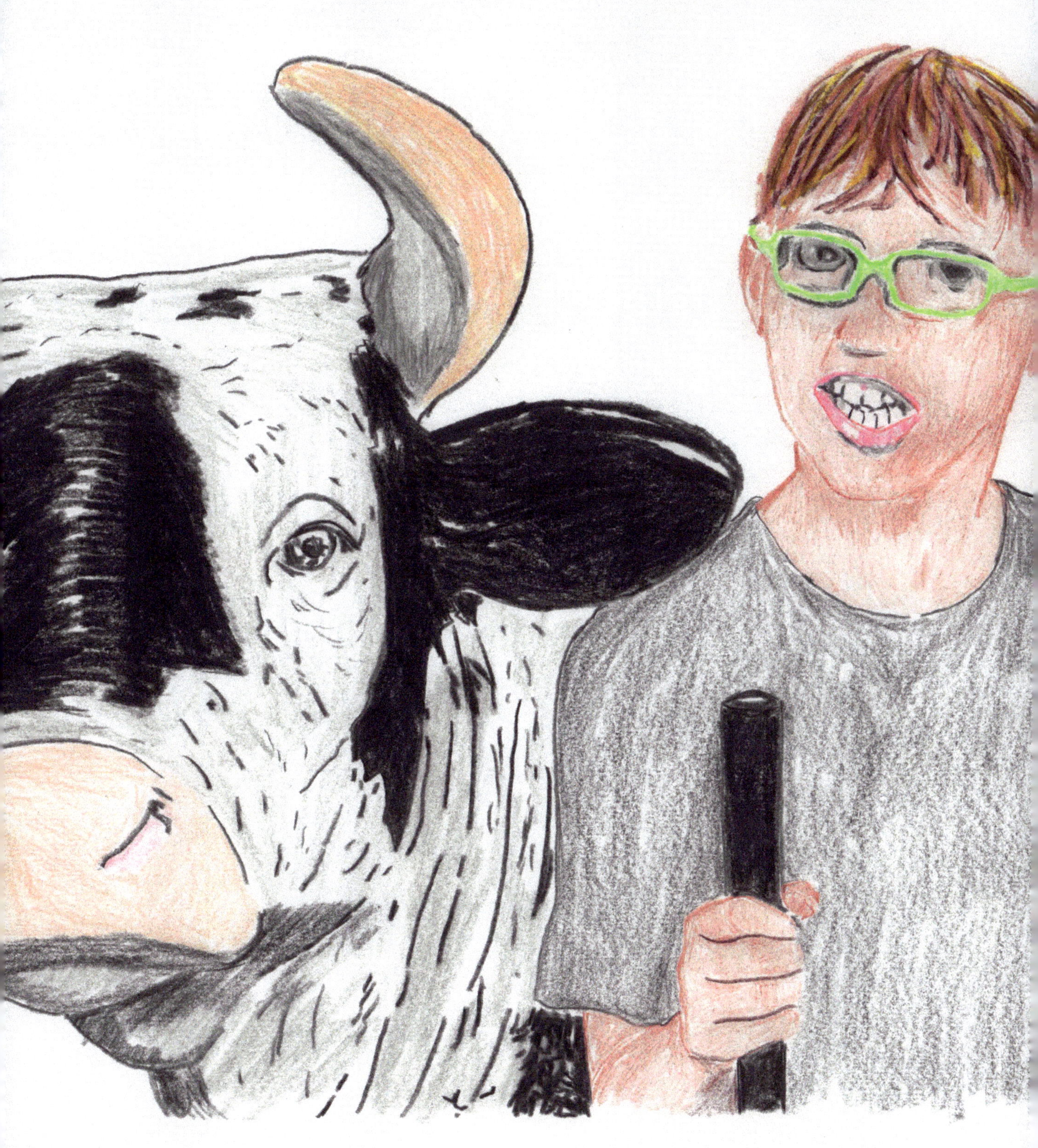

You are so much fun, you are smart, and caring too. If all that makes you weird, then I want to be weird like you.

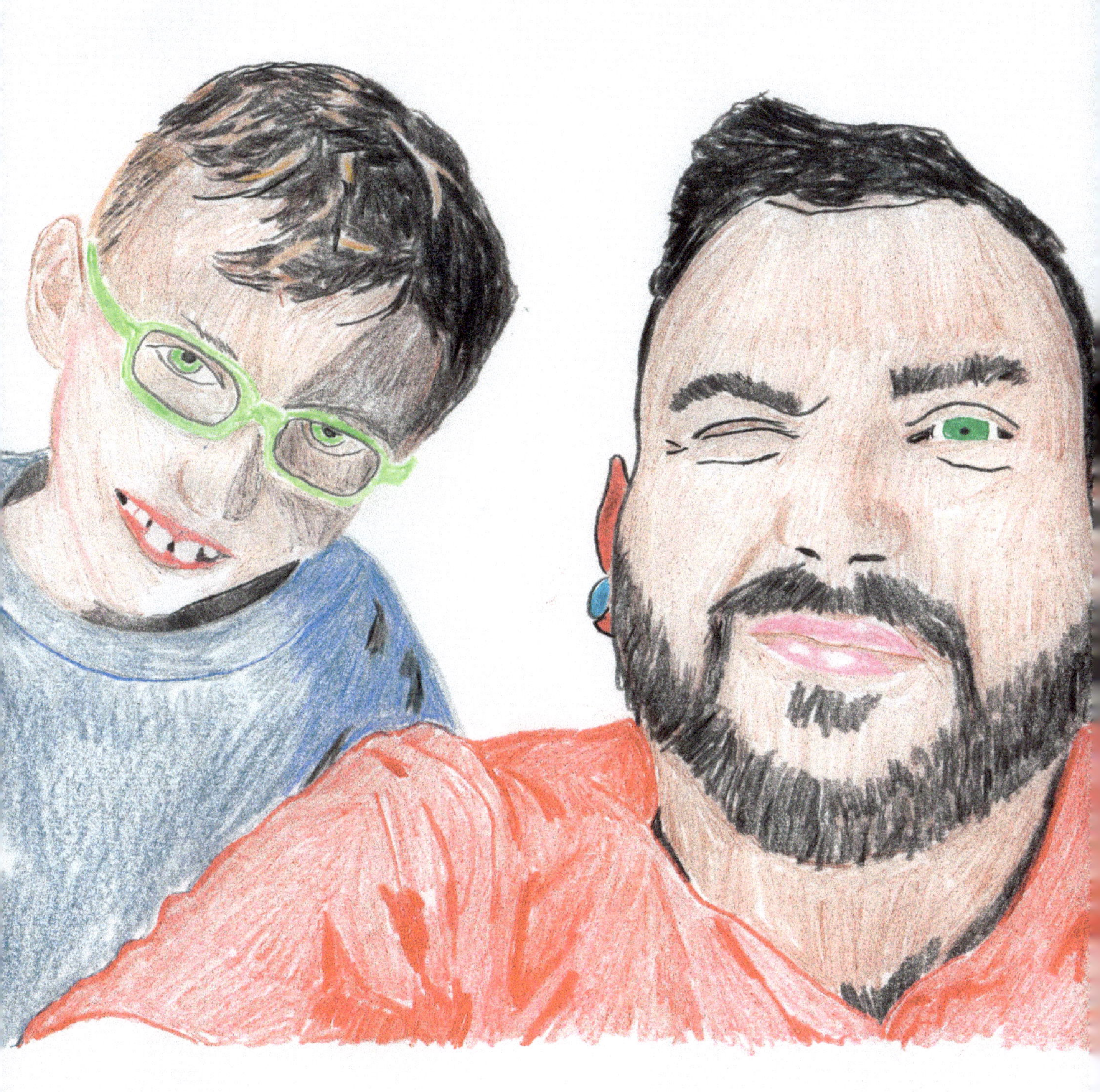